Diets to help
MIGRAINE

MARTIN BUDD

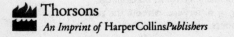

Thorsons
An Imprint of HarperCollins*Publishers*

Thorsons
An Imprint of HarperCollins*Publishers*
77–85 Fulham Palace Road,
Hammersmith, London W6 8JB
1160 Battery Street
San Francisco, California 94111–1213

Published by Thorsons 1997
10 9 8 7 6 5 4 3 2 1

Martin Budd asserts the moral right to
be identified as the author of this work

A catalogue record for this book
is available from the British Library

ISBN 0 7225 3326 8

Printed in Great Britain by
Caledonian International Book Manufacturing Ltd, Glasgow

Contents

Introduction

The connection between food and drink and migraine attacks has been known about for a very long time. Many migraine sufferers (or *migraineurs*, as they are called in America) are well aware that specific foods or drinks can trigger their migraine attack, and much work and research has been done to identify and understand the role of these 'trigger foods'.

This concept of allergy foods and migraine is not new. Back in 1905 Dr Francis Hare observed that incompatible foods could cause a headache.

If a link between specific foods and migraine symptoms can be established, then avoidance of such foods should lead to relief from the migraine. But unfortunately establishing the link is not always easy. The response to a suspect food leading to symptoms can be anything from 10 minutes to 36 hours! This time difference is determined by absorption speed and efficiency in the body system, and gut transit time.

NON-FOOD 'TRIGGERS'

To add to this confusion there are also many well defined non-food triggers. These include: hormone factors (PMS), time of day, fatigue, missed meals, inappropriate or excessive exercise, and neck or spinal injury or misuse, that may influence the blood circulation to the head. Even the type of pillow or pillows we use in bed can be significant. Work-related strains and emotional stress are also factors.

In addition, many migraines that are not linked to specific foods fall under the umbrella of *hypoglycaemic migraines*. These are headaches caused by sudden swings in the blood sugar – either a rapid speed of fall in the sugar or a chronic low level of blood sugar. These hypoglycaemic headaches will be discussed fully in later chapters.

MIXED TRIGGER MIGRAINES

There are approximately five million migraine sufferers in the UK, and although I have regularly treated people with this problem for over 30 years, I have yet to see two patients with identical trigger patterns and symptoms. The combination of various trigger factors and the great variety of symptoms appear to be almost endless.

It seems likely that many migraine patients only develop their symptoms when several triggers occur at the same time, creating the concept of 'mixed trigger migraines'. An example could be a migraine that only develops for a woman after a weekend lie-in, following a late or missed breakfast, this occurring just prior to a period. Not surprisingly, these mixed triggers only occur infrequently, and this could explain why some people only have a migraine once or twice a year!

THE IMPORTANCE OF GOOD NUTRITION

Although non-food triggers are discussed, this book is mainly concerned with describing the ideal diet to minimize the frequency and severity of migraine headaches. I have found that, while hormonal, structural, emotional and other causes may be present, the *central* element in migraine treatment is correct nutrition. However, simply avoiding certain trigger foods is not always the answer. This may provide some symptom relief, however migraine is not simply a headache but a whole body imbalance. A susceptibility to migraine, that may run through a family, is not likely to be resolved by simply avoiding cheese or chocolate.

With this in mind, migraine sufferers who follow the advice offered should improve in general health in addition to headache relief. This offers a valuable first step to minimize the symptoms of a debilitating and depressing condition.

CHAPTER ONE

What Happens During a Migraine Attack?

Most of us think of pain as having its origin in the nerves. Whether the cause is infection, damage or simple pressure, we usually assume that pain develops as a result of irritation to a nerve or nerves. But the symptoms of a migraine attack do not fit into this explanation, because migraine symptoms are caused by changes in the blood volume within the brain. A migraine headache is a *vascular* headache. Other examples of vascular pain include cramp, angina, temporal arteritis and Raynaud's phenomena. (Vascular meaning, vessels for conveying blood.)

The nerves do play a part in pain transmission and awareness, but the essential component of migraine is an initial reduction in blood to the brain, followed by an overswing in compensation and increase in the blood volume, causing the familiar head pain and other symptoms.

During a migraine attack there are two well-defined stages:

- **Stage 1**
  At the beginning, following one or more triggers (discussed later), the blood vessels throughout the body become narrowed or constricted; this is known as vaso-constriction. The effect of this vaso-constriction on the brain causes the pre-headache symptoms familiar to many migraine sufferers. These include photophobia (i.e. intolerance of light), dizziness, nausea, feeling chilled etc.

- **Stage 2**
  The body's metabolism responds to the reduction in blood supply by compensating with an expansion or dilation of the blood vessels; this is known as vaso-dilation. Unfortunately, as often occurs with the body's back-up systems, there is an overswing and too *much* blood dilates the blood vessels – causing pain and headaches.

SEROTONIN

A compound found in the blood called serotonin plays a major role in these two stages of migraine. This substance, an amine derived from the amino acid *tryptophan*, is a neurotransmitter or 'chemical messenger'. It facilitates with the transmission of nerve impulses from cell to cell. Around 98 per cent of the serotonin in our blood can be found in the platelets. These minute cells in the blood bind together in response to tissue damage to assist blood clotting. When this occurs, the serotonin is released from the platelets – causing contraction of the surrounding blood vessels and thus minimizing blood loss.

This leads to two important questions:

1 Even when there is no actual tissue damage and/or bleeding, why do the platelets release serotonin during a migraine attack, when it is not really needed? (And why is the whole body involved in this reaction?)

2 When the platelets clump together during the first stage of a migraine attack, are actual blood clots formed?

It is thought that substances known as **vaso-active amines**, found in certain foods and drinks, cause the platelets to stick together. In non-migraineurs this is prevented by the body releasing protective enzymes. The chief of these is monoamine oxidase (which gives its name to the MOA inhibitor drugs). These enzymes, which are probably deficient in the blood of migraine sufferers, act by breaking down or reducing the potency of the vaso-active amines. Fortunately, although there is a tendency for the platelets to release serotonin, under the conditions discussed above, no actual clotting occurs. It would seem that our metabolism recognizes the absence of tissue damage and blood loss.

High levels of serotonin occur shortly after eating vaso-active amines in food, but low levels can result from stress, low blood sugar and a fall in blood oestrogen, as occurs in menstruation. Inappropriate and sudden low levels of serotonin can lead to the increase in blood volume as described above in Stage 2.

Many drugs prescribed for migraine act by increasing the serotonin levels, producing vaso-construction. These include caffeine, ergotomine-based drugs and the beta-blockers. Prescribing drugs to increase serotonin may seem a paradox, when increased serotonin (as in Stage 1) causes the migraine. Although the serotonin initially causes a reduction in blood flow, the drugs are, in fact, prescribed to achieve the same effect, but these are targeted to treat the over-compensated vaso-dilation that is a characteristic of Stage 2, and actually is responsible for the migraine headaches.

It should be remembered that vaso-constriction followed by a compensatory vaso-dilation, with an increase in the blood volume to the brain, is the dominant characteristic of many of the food trigger causes of migraine (whether vaso-active amine specific, or allergy caused or as a response to low blood sugar).

HOW DO FOODS TRIGGER MIGRAINES?

The physical and chemical changes that occur in the head when migraineurs eat certain foods is still not fully understood. For many years, researchers and physicians have worked to identify a recognizable pattern of cause and effect with food-triggered migraines. However, as human beings we are all unique and there is no such condition as a 'typical' migraine.

Nevertheless, it has been generally agreed that there are two well-defined groups of food triggers. These are:

1 Vaso-active trigger foods
2 Food allergy triggers.

To these I would like to add a further category of food triggers:

3 Hypoglycaemia (low blood sugar) triggers.

This can all sound rather confusing, particularly as there is a degree of overlapping within the three groups, and many migraines are caused by multiple triggers. So I will try now to identify the special characteristics of the three trigger groups and the specific role of each in causing migraine symptoms.

1 VASO-ACTIVE TRIGGER FOODS

This group comprises the foods and drinks that many of us usually associate with migraines. These triggers all contain vaso-active substances known as amines (protein components). They cause changes in the blood chemistry and an eventual increase in blood volume to the brain – along with headaches and other symptoms.

The best known amine is **histamine**. Found chiefly in alcohol, it produces symptoms by changing the blood brain barrier permeability and allowing other amines to influence the circulation.

The food amines include tyramine, phenylethylamine, synephrine, and octopamine. When these substances are consumed in our food and drink, they do not of course automatically give everyone a migraine. But it seems likely that those of us who lack the protective enzyme **monoamine oxidase** are prone to migraine symptoms.

Other amines involved in the cause and the treatment of migraine include the catecholamines. These include adrenalin, dopamine and nor-adrenalin. This group is formed from the amino acids phenylalamine and tyrosine.

Vaso-active amines

The main vaso-active amines and the foods and drinks in which they are found are listed below:

- *Tyramine*
  Contained in cheese (particularly the blue and matured varieties, but much smaller amounts in Brie and Camembert, and only a negligible amount in cottage cheese), potatoes (small amounts only) and smoked fish. (Decaying gut bacteria also contains tyramine.)
- *Histamine*
  Contained in alcohol.
- *Phenylethylamine*
  Contained in chocolate (plain more than milk), and cocoa.
- *Synephrine*
  Contained in citrus fruit; the juices contain more than the whole fruit.

- *Octopamine*
  Contained in citrus fruit, pips and skins.

Other vaso-active substances that are not amines include monosodium glutamate, caffeine and aspartane.

2 FOOD ALLERGY TRIGGERS

Many migraine sufferers blame the 'three Cs' for their symptoms. These include cheese, chocolate, and the citrus fruits and juices. In addition, red wine is a frequent culprit. As previously discussed, these all contain the vaso-active amines that can cause circulation changes within the brain and eventual headaches and other symptoms. However, although up to 80 per cent of migraine patients are sensitive to specific foods and drinks, many specialists treating food allergies do *not* agree that the three Cs and wine cause the majority of migraines.

This view is supported by evidence which confirms that elimination of the vaso-active amine foods and drinks only actually prevents migraine in two to three per cent of cases. A report in *The Lancet* (October 1983) showed that in a selected group of 88 schoolchildren, who all suffered regular and severe migraines, 93 per cent recovered and became virtually symptom-free after following a low-risk, limited food, elimination diet (or oligo-antigenic diet).

Aside from the specific role of the vaso-active amines (previously discussed) the exact manner in which allergies cause migraine symptoms is not fully understood. However, we know that allergic reactions can lead to fluid retention or oedema in tissue. It is quite possible that an allergic brain reaction may cause swelling and pressure against the inside of the skull. This could produce the severe throbbing headache associated with migraine attacks.

3 FOOD TRIGGERS AND LOW BLOOD SUGAR

The main types of migraine attacks that are linked to low blood sugar include:

1 High sugar diets and migraine
2 Pre-menstrual migraines
3 Missed meal migraines
4 The 'weekend' migraine
5 Migraines following exercise
6 Stress migraines

In these cases low blood sugar can lead to changes in the blood volume to the brain, with vasodilation (bulging) of the blood vessels within the brain and subsequent headaches and other symptoms.

CHAPTER TWO

Migraines and Food Triggers

As we have seen in Chapter 1, there are three main groups of food-based migraine triggers. These are:

1 foods that contain vaso-active amines, such as chocolate, cheese and alcohol
2 foods which you have an allergy to, for example, wheat, milk, tomatoes
3 a high-sugar diet that can predispose to low blood sugar.

It must be stated at this point that not all migraines are food triggered. There are many migraine sufferers who have never linked their symptoms to food or drink. Although not caused by specific foods, migraines can be triggered by changes in the blood sugar and other factors already mentioned (hormonal factors, stress etc.).

With this in mind it is worthwhile identifying which trigger group applies to your symptoms, always remembering that the three groups frequently overlap. I have seen migraine patients who react to the amine-rich foods, experience reactions because of specific food allergies *and* also have low blood sugar. Fortunately, there is usually a dominant trigger and this should be identified as a first step. There are certain diagnostic clues which can help to pinpoint your particular food triggers. Each of the three groups has a characteristic 'symptom-picture' in terms of timing, intensity, variety and frequency in relation to food eaten.

We will now look at each of these groups in turn.

1 VASO-ACTIVE AMINE TRIGGERS

For many migraine sufferers, this group contains the most easily identifiable food triggers. It includes citrus fruits, cheese, chocolate etc., as looked at in more detail in Chapter 1.

The chain of events that can be triggered by consuming these foods or drinks is usually rapid. Although the 'transit time' for a meal to pass through our digestive tract can be up to three days, most migraineurs tend to react to their offending food in a matter of two or three hours or sooner. The actual amount of quantity of food eaten is not a relevant factor. I have heard of migraines which continued for six or seven days with vomiting, headache and photophobia, after eating just one square of chocolate! Therefore many people who react badly to the vaso-active rich foods learn quickly to recognize the foods and drinks which cause their symptoms and to avoid them.

The degree of tolerance – or rather intolerance – to such foods can vary, but strict avoidance of known triggers is usually worthwhile as many sufferers can then remain virtually migraine-free. (This only occurs, of course, in the absence of triggers from the other groups.)

The link between the amine-rich foods and drinks and migraine is not too difficult to establish, making this group perhaps the easiest of the three to treat successfully with a minimum amount of disruption to a person's diet.

2 FOOD ALLERGY TRIGGERS

Unfortunately it is not always so easy to deal with the foods in this second group. Many physicians treating migraine consider that the effects of the amine-rich foods have been grossly exaggerated, and that actual food allergies – which constitute the largest group of triggers – cause a far greater number of migraines. Unfortunately, unlike the reactions to chocolate, alcohol and cheese etc., food allergies are often hidden or masked. The list of foods that are implicated as allergens in migraine attacks is huge and includes most of the commonly eaten foods. (See list below.) The key to understanding allergies, particularly multiple or masked allergies, lies in the fact that allergic reactions usually occur only when a food is eaten repeatedly. Many migraine sufferers have identified a 'build-up' factor with their reaction to specific foods. In other words, the symptoms only develop after the same food has been eaten on three or four consecutive days. (This type of delayed allergic response highlights the value of the five to seven-day rotation diet. See page 28.)

The commonest migraine-causing allergen foods include wheat, cows' milk, coffee, pork, yeast, eggs and tomatoes. However, trials have shown that some individuals have multiple allergies involving a sensitivity to more than 25 different foods and drinks.

Allergies fall into two groups: **fixed allergies**, which are often from birth and do not usually cease with time; and **temporary allergies**, which are more easily treated, and tolerance of a particular food or drink can often be re-established after three or four months of avoidance.

Food Groups and Families

If there is an allergy to a particular food, it is important at the beginning also to avoid the other foods in the same food family. These families are listed in Appendix A on page 74.

Foods known to provoke migraine
(Listed in order of percentage)

Foods	%
Cows' milk	63
Wheat	50
Chocolate	46
Egg	35
Orange	32
Cheese	32
Tomato	23
Rye	22

Foods	%
Rice	22
Shellfish	22
Grapes	22
Onions	21
Soya	21
Pork	19
Peanut	19
Alcohol	18
Walnut	18
Beef	17
Tea	17
Coffee	17
Goats' milk	16
Corn (maize)	15
Oats	15
Sugar (cane)	13
Yeast	13
Apple	12
Potato	12
Chicken	11
Banana	7
Strawberry	6

This list is compiled from four trials on migraine and food allergies. The top 30 offending foods are listed according to frequency. Therefore cows' milk sensitivity occurred with 63 per cent of the migraineurs and wheat occurred with 50 per cent and so on. It is interesting to note that the only vegetables listed are onions, tomatoes and potatoes. The only major cereal not on the list is barley, but the absence of many game meats, poultry, fish and lamb provides for plenty of choice when designing a limited food diet. Remember that goat's milk and goat's milk yogurt and cheese can be seen as 'safer' than cows' milk products, as can sheep's milk and its products.

Food Allergy Testing

There are many different procedures to test for suspect foods (assuming that simple avoidance has not identified the culprits), which range from pulse testing to blood testing. These are discussed in detail in Chapter 3.

3 SUGAR TRIGGERS AND LOW BLOOD SUGAR

This last group of triggers does not involve specific foods, but implicates the role of sugar-rich foods in causing migraine. Unlike the allergy triggers, very little nutritional detective work is needed to recognize the role of low blood sugar as a migraine trigger. Although the consumption of sugar and sugar-rich food provides clues to understanding and diagnosing this problem, the timing of meals, food avoidance, stress, exercise, our hormones and several other factors, all play a part. (See Chapter 4 for a detailed explanation of the blood sugar connection.)

CHAPTER THREE

The Diagnosis of Food Triggers

Having identified and discussed the three main groups of food triggers in migraine, it would now be helpful to find out which group is responsible for *your* migraine and, if possible, to work out which actual foods cause symptoms.

Therefore this chapter deals with the many and varied diagnostic tests used to reveal the food triggers.

1 VASO-ACTIVE AMINE-RICH FOODS AND DRINKS

The amine-rich foods are fortunately few in number. They include cheese (particularly mature blue cheeses), smoked fish, potatoes, alcohol, chocolate, cocoa, citrus fruit and citrus fruit juice. There is rarely a need to test for these foods and drinks with migraine sufferers because, if they react to the amines, the cause and effect is predictable and obvious. Very few foods are involved, and the symptoms develop rapidly and predictably –

leaving very little room to doubt the nature of the trigger substance.

Unlike the many and varied foods and drinks that are included in the next section on allergies, the amine-rich foods are easily identified and usually wisely avoided. The symptom-relief obtained confirms which foods are culprits. I find that some patients *only* experience a full-blown migraine when they inadvertently consume some chocolate or cheese, for example, which is normally taboo for them. (See Appendix C on page 82 for details of substitute-foods to eat instead.)

2 ALLERGIES

Allergy testing is a vast and complex subject, and this book is mainly concerned with the dietary treatment of migraine. However, it may be helpful to list briefly the various testing methods in use.

Allergy testing for migraine and other symptoms falls into two broad categories. These are: laboratory tests and non-laboratory tests.

Laboratory Tests

Although these tests have some limitations and drawbacks, they are well proven and generally predictable and diagnostically useful. They can, however, be expensive. A list of the main types of tests follows, with brief comments on their value and accuracy:

- *Skin scratch testing*
  Essentially a measurement of skin response, which may be negative in the presence of a general allergy, this is seen by many specialists as being only 50 per cent accurate.

- *FICA – Food Immune Complex Assay (IgE testing)*
  Involves the measurement of blood antibodies that increase with allergic foods. Unfortunately there are people who tend to show high levels of these blood antibodies (IgE's) but who do not show allergic tendencies or symptoms.

- *Cytotoxic testing*
  Also a blood test, involving an assessment of white cell changes. A costly test, difficult to replicate. The results depend largely on the technician's skill and judgement for their accuracy, and are thus considered unreliable.

- *RAST testing (Radio-allergo-sorbent test)*
  A complex and expensive blood test, similar in principle to the FICA test. Fundamentally unreliable, as localized reactions do not necessarily reflect in blood changes.

- *ELISA (Enzyme Linked Immunosorbent Assay)*
  A costly but very accurate blood test. Laboratories claim 75 per cent accuracy. Ideal for food allergies. Only one small blood sample is required to test for over 90 foods.

- *Provocation–Neutralization testing*
  Minute amounts of foods are injected under the skin or placed under the tongue. Similar to the homoeopathic 'like cures like' principle, foods that provoke

can also neutralize symptoms. Injecting can cause severe allergic reactions, however, and false positives can occur with this type of testing.

Non-Laboratory Tests

These include the use of special apparatus or specific diagnostic testing:

- *EAV (Electro-Acupuncture or Vega testing)*
  This test measures the skin's electrical activity at designated acupuncture points. A galvanometer is used and it provides a useful and speedy first step to assessing food and environmental allergies. No needles are involved which makes it ideal for testing children.

- *A/K testing (Applied Kinesiology)*
  Those who use AK claim that foods can adversely influence the strength of specific muscles. This is a controversial technique that relies very heavily on the operator's skill and protocol, which can lead to a lack of standardisation and accuracy.

- *Coca Pulse testing*
  This simple test is based on pulse-rate increases with allergic foods. Although a little tedious, this test can be used at home. The radial pulse is checked at 20, 40, 60, 80 and 100 minutes after eating single foods. This offers a simple self-check for suspect foods.

- *Fasting and Exclusion Diet testing*
  In addition to the pulse testing, there are two other types of food provocation challenge testing that can be carried out at home, which are: fasting, followed

by food reintroduction, and exclusion diet (or limited food or rare food), followed by food reintroduction. Both these methods are designed to achieve a symptom-free condition by avoiding the foods of suspected of being allergens. This is done either by total food avoidance or by eating rare or 'safe' foods. Testing to identify particular allergy foods is the second stage and is achieved by systematic food reintroduction or challenge.

We will now look at each of these methods in more detail.

FASTING

This is a controversial procedure which involves food avoidance for five days and drinking only glass-bottled mineral water. Our metabolism reacts to a complete fast in many ways, including fat breakdown and changes in the blood sugar. Any withdrawal symptoms usually occur within the initial 48 hours.

Discipline and care are required for a five-day fast. Underweight and seriously ill patients are excluded. It is not considered appropriate to test those who suffer severe reactions to foods, and asthmatic and epileptic patients are also excluded. Alkaline salts may be prescribed to clear the bowels.

After the fast, and assuming there is symptom relief, selected foods are introduced individually and any symptoms are noted. In addition to symptom assessment, some testers see a diagnostic value in observing changes in the handwriting and pulse-rate. All such reactions to the reintroduction of foods after the fast are seen as diagnostically significant.

EXCLUSION DIETS

This logical and effective procedure involves following a diet that excludes all the foods which commonly trigger migraine attacks. It is called the *oliogo-antigenic diet* or limited food diet. If the migraineur does *not* have a migraine when following this diet, it can safely be assumed that food plays a major role in causing the symptoms. Conversely, if *no* symptom relief occurs, then factors other than food must be involved in triggering the migraines.

A big drawback when manipulating the diet in this way (i.e. using it as a diagnostic tool), is the difficulty in assessing results if the pattern of a person's migraine is only three or four attacks each year. However, with such infrequent episodes, a food trigger factor is unlikely to be the prime cause. Therefore exclusion diets are better carried out only by those who suffer regular and predictable attacks (for example, at least twice monthly).

The Lancet trial

In 1983 *The Lancet* carried details of a comprehensive controlled trial to identify the role of food sensitivity in causing frequent or severe migraines in children. It may be useful to look closely at this report in order to understand the value of this type of testing.

The results showed that 93 per cent of the children recovered after following a limited food diet for three to four weeks. The method used to identify allergic foods fell into two stages: limited food and reintroduction.

- *Stage 1: Limited food (oligo-antigenic diet)*
  This diet consisted of one food from each of the following food groups:

  Meat: Lamb or chicken.
  Vegetables: Any brassica (mustard family). This includes cabbage, kale, swede, turnip, kohlrabi, cauliflower, Brussels sprouts and broccoli.
  Carbohydrate: Rice or potato.
  Fruit: Banana or apple.
  Drinks: Mineral water only (glass-bottled).

  The children who followed this diet were selected on the basis of suffering at *least* one migraine each week over the previous six months. Other causes of headaches were ruled out. These included middle-ear disease, dental problems, high blood-pressure etc. Participants were included in the trial on the basis of suffering regular migraine headaches, plus *two* other associated symptoms, which included facial pallor, photophobia, giddiness, nausea etc.

- *Stage 2: Food reintroduction*
  If *no* headaches, or only one, occurred during the

final two weeks of the four-week diet, food was reintroduced. In the event that a child did *not* experience symptom relief, a second limited food diet was prescribed, which excluded all the foods that the child had eaten on the initial diet.

Those children who became symptom-free after the four-week trial were allowed to eat a daily helping of excluded foods, at the rate of *one* food per seven days. These foods then became a regular part of the diet, but were again excluded if symptoms (i.e. headaches), were provoked. Foods were in this way introduced systematically until the diet was 'nutritionally and socially acceptable'.

Eighty-eight children completed the initial exclusion diet. Of these, six showed no improvement and 78 recovered completely, being symptom-free. Significantly, after the introduction of additional foods, after the fifth week, 74 children relapsed and their symptoms returned.

The reintroduction of foods was determined by family habits and individual taste, allowing for considerable flexibility. It was interesting to note that although one of the children showed a reaction to 24 foods, he was still able to follow a nutritionally acceptable diet, whilst at the same time avoiding the foods that caused symptoms. He remained symptom-free.

A total of 55 different foods provoked symptoms in the 74 children who relapsed after the fifth week. The 10 main culprits are listed below:

Food etc.	Children affected
Cows' milk	27
Eggs	24
Chocolate	22
Orange	21
Wheat	21
Benzoic acid (*see below*)	14
Cheese (cows' milk)	13
Tomato	13
Tartrazine (*see below*)	12
Rye	12

Benzoic acid (E210) This is used as a preservative in food; it is also an antibacterial and anti-fungal agent, which occurs naturally in certain edible berries, but it is usually synthetically manufactured. It can be found in the following foodstuffs: jams, beers, sweet sauces and syrups, fruit juice and purees, pickles, salad creams, pickled herrings and mackerel, fruit yogurts and coffee essence.

Tartrazine (E102) This notorious additive is a yellow-coloured azo-dye. It can be found in many orange or yellow-coloured convenience foods, including: sweets, cakes, biscuits, smoked cod, haddock and herrings, lemon and lime drinks, sea food dressings, mint jelly and sauce, salad cream, fruit pies, and pie fillings, marzipan, piccalilli, brown sauce, tinned processed peas, soft drinks, and coloured pill coatings.

Processed Foods and Allergies

A common factor occurring in many trials carried out to identify food allergies and sensitivities is processed food. The more the food is processed, the more likely it is to provoke a reaction. Food chemistry can be altered by almost every stage of food processing and storage or preserving. An example of this is the proven fact that many people react to white flour products but not wholemeal flour products. Some symptoms are triggered by eating pork but many more are produced by eating bacon.

It is worth noting that in the 'top 10' list identified in *The Lancet* trial, two of the substances were food additives (see above). As these are found in many foods, it is very important when following a simple, minimal food diet to avoid processed foods of *all* types. (A little research will also help to identify the additives in the same chemical family, for example Tartrazine is an azo dye; the other azo dyes include E107, E110, E122, E123, E124, E128, E151, E180 and 154 and 155 and they are also worth avoiding.) It is also advisable to avoid tinned and frozen foods completely and to wash fruit and vegetables thoroughly.

When following the initial exclusion diet in an attempt to achieve symptom relief, it is also essential to avoid known environmental triggers. These include smokey atmospheres, aerosol sprays, perfumes, aftershaves and deodorants and plastic water bottles. It is important to remember that an allergy to a particular fruit or vegetable usually means that the other members of the same family may also give rise to symptoms. (See Appendix A on page 74.)

ROTATION DIETS

The well-designed *Lancet* trial, outlined above, drew attention to several other important considerations when carrying out a restricted food test diet.

The *average* time lapse between eating a food and the provoking symptoms is two days. But the full time range, from eating to the onset of symptoms, can be from one hour up to seven days. This suggests that a rotation diet, which has been advocated for those who are very sensitive to new food allergens, should ideally be on a seven day, and not a four or five day, basis.

Although the simplest and most obvious way of dealing with food allergies is the complete avoidance of the culprit foods, a seven-day rotation diet can avoid build-up allergies and allow for recovery time if the allergic response is not too severe. With any rotation diet it is important not to eat members of the same fruit or vegetable family on consecutive days. Some allergy specialists maintain that foods of the same family can be eaten every *other* day; for example, it would be possible to have cabbage on Monday, broccoli on Wednesday and cauliflower on Friday. These are all in the mustard family and should not be eaten on consecutive days. Rotation diets are prescribed to allow time for our systems to recover from the effects of specific foods before we eat them again.

3 LOW BLOOD SUGAR (HYPOGLYCAEMIA)

The diagnosis of low blood sugar plays a very important role in assessing and identifying migraine food triggers. The most useful test to identify low blood sugar as a potential trigger is the six-hour glucose tolerance test.

The Glucose Tolerance Test (GTT)

The Glucose Tolerance Test is the most reliable and informative test for functional hypoglycaemia. The duration of the test should be six hours, although two-hour and five-hour tests are also frequently requested. The two-hour test is essentially a test for diabetes and it is virtually useless to diagnose hypoglycaemia. The six-hour test is to be preferred to a five-hour test. The nadir (lowest level) and the adrenal compensation towards the end of the test are more likely to be seen in the six-hour test.

In order to carry out the test, the patient is requested to fast on water for 12 to 14 hours (usually overnight) and an early blood sugar measurement is made. Blood can be taken from the arm for a laboratory test, or a finger prick glucometer test can be used. After this 'fasting' test, 50g of soluble glucose are given to the patient to drink in approximately 300ml (½ pint) water. Further blood sugar checks are made at the following times after drinking the glucose:

50g glucose
Sample 2 – 30 minutes
Sample 3 – 60 minutes
Sample 4 – 120 minutes
Sample 5 – 180 minutes
Sample 6 – 270 minutes
Sample 7 – 360 minutes

The blood sugar will increase after taking the glucose but, if the sugar control mechanism is working normally, the blood sugar will return to the same level as the fasting level. If diabetes is present the blood sugar will be too high throughout the test.

With reactive or functional hypoglycaemia there is usually an excessive insulin response to the glucose drink and, after an initial rise, the blood sugar level falls to a low point, often 30 to 40 per cent lower than the fasting level. This inappropriate and sudden fall in the blood sugar triggers an adrenal compensation and adrenalin is released to raise the blood sugar.

All this information is available from the test results, but a full six-hour test is needed and a single fasting sample (which is usually quite normal), does not show anything diagnostically useful. Hypoglycaemia is thought to be caused either by an insulin excess (*hyperinsulinism*) or an adrenal deficiency (*hypoadrenalism*). Both of these disorders can be identified on a GTT graph.

Although this test confirms a general tendency to low blood sugar after taking glucose, the pattern of symptoms in terms of time of day and time of month (as discussed in Chapter 1) is also diagnostically valuable. In my practice I frequently loan a glucometer to patients to carry out their own finger-prick blood glucose checks over an extended period of time, and particularly when the headaches occur. These results frequently provide confirmation of a link between inappropriately low blood sugar levels and the symptoms of migraine.

Hypoglycaemia or Allergy?

I believe that many migraine sufferers have multiple triggers which cause their symptoms. When this is suspected it is advisable to eliminate the triggers one at a time. A useful starting point is to diagnose (or eliminate) any tendency to hypoglycaemia. Many patients, who have for several years identified certain foods as migraine triggers, have often found to their delight that when their blood sugar is stable they can eat the culprit foods without developing symptoms.

As an osteopath also I always attempt to normalize the neck structure and movement, and again this frequently allows previous 'food triggers' to be eaten with impunity.

CHAPTER FOUR

The Blood Sugar Connection

BACKGROUND

For more than seventy years the link between low blood sugar and migraine has been studied by doctors and nutritionists.

Insulin-dependent diabetics experience difficulty at times in precisely assessing their insulin needs. This can lead them to overdosing inadvertently, causing hyper-insulinism and low blood sugar (hypoglycaemia), which is termed the 'hypo' effect. When this sudden and inappropriate fall in the blood sugar occurs, the body compensates with a release of adrenalin from the paired adrenal glands. It is this surge of adrenalin that causes many of the 'hypo' symptoms, including breathlessness, palpitations, headaches, sweating and fatigue.

In the early 1920s, a contemporary of Banting and Best (the co-discoverers of insulin), observed that some of his non-diabetic patients were also experiencing 'hypo' symptoms similar to diabetics. Dr Seale Harris, an American GP, presented his ideas in 1924, in the *Journal of the American Medical Association*. In doing so he drew attention to a little understood medical condition that has been a subject of some controversy to this day.

Dr Harris suggested that many non-diabetic patients with symptoms of low blood sugar suffered as a result of overactivity of the insulin-producing glands of the pancreas. This overactivity is caused in many cases by a high sugar diet, so leading to hyperinsulinism and low blood sugar. The name for this condition is *reactive* or *functional hypoglycaemia*.

Dr Harris argued that many glands of the body can become hyperactive as a result of excessive stimulation, and that this overactivity may be followed by metabolic exhaustion and underactivity. This logical concept explains why hyperthyroidism often precedes hypothyroidism and why many late-onset diabetics have a previous history of low blood sugar.

To put it in simple terms: too much insulin with low blood sugar may be followed by an eventual gland deficiency with too little insulin and diabetes (high blood sugar). You may be thinking at this stage that this is all very interesting but what does it have to do with migraine? The answer is there is a great deal of evidence to prove that a strong causal link exists between low blood sugar and migraine headaches. Many practitioners and researchers believe that food intolerance or actual food allergies can trigger migraine attacks, but another cause is frequently an inappropriate low level of blood sugar. I also believe this is the case and I shall describe in this book a comprehensive and effective dietary programme to treat low blood sugar and migraines caused by low blood sugar.

Migraine and Diabetes

An interesting confirmation of the role of low blood sugar in causing migraine lies in the relationship of migraine to diabetes. As we know, in diabetes there is an excess of sugar in the blood. Therefore, if *low* blood sugar contributes to migraines, why do diabetics also experience migraine? The answer is that far fewer diabetics have migraine than do non-diabetics. In this context, diabetes is thought to play a 'protective' role in migraine. When diabetics suffer migraines, it is commonly in the early hours, when they are particularly prone to low blood sugar episodes.

There are many instances where chronic migraine sufferers find to their delight that they are experiencing fewer headaches as they reach mid-life. Their delight is subdued, however, when they are diagnosed as having late-onset diabetes. There are many other examples to highlight the common link between low blood sugar and migraine. These are outlined below.

PRE-MENSTRUAL AND MENOPAUSAL MIGRAINE

Pre-menstrual syndrome (PMS) can include some or all of the following symptoms: fluid retention, fatigue, mood swings, headaches, sugar craving, nausea and temperature changes. These symptoms, which usually occur in women aged from 15 to 50 years, can also be present during the menopause, however. The chief reason for these symptoms is a fall in the level of the female hormone oestrogen.

Statistically, around 60 per cent of female migraine sufferers claim that their menstrual cycle influences their symptoms. Significantly the blood sugar level falls for three to four days before periods, and pre-menstrual migraines are often accompanied by sugar cravings.

MISSED MEAL MIGRAINES

In a recent comprehensive survey of migraine in school-children (*British Medical Journal*, September 1994), carried out at the Royal Aberdeen Children's Hospital, it was concluded that the prevalence of migraine in schoolchildren is approximately 11 per cent. One of the co-authors of this survey, Dr Geary Russel, stated that the *main* trigger factor in childhood migraine was missed meals.

We know that our blood sugar normally begins to fall two to three hours after eating a meal. If a meal is missed, the resulting low blood sugar may precipitate a migraine. This phenomenon is particularly apparent when breakfast is missed. For all of us, the blood sugar normally falls to a low point between 3 and 4 a.m. (This is a time when many migraines develop.) It follows that if a migraine sufferer avoids eating for 14 to 18 hours as a result of missing breakfast, he or she will become particularly vulnerable to a migraine attack in the middle of the morning.

Significantly, for many years fasting has been used as a predictable method of creating a migraine attack for research purposes. It seems likely that the fatigue, stress and haste so often associated with missed meals are also contributing factors.

THE WEEKEND MIGRAINE

Many migraine sufferers experience weekend head-aches. There is understandable annoyance and frustration when, after a headache-free busy working week, a migraine attack develops after a weekend lie-in. Here is the same cause and effect as in the missed meal or missed breakfast headaches. The resulting low blood sugar leads to the migraine with the over-long gap between meals.

THE EXERCISE TRIGGER

Many migraines are triggered by exercise or sport. This is not too surprising as we know that both these activities have the potential to reduce the blood sugar. This happens either because the exercise has used up the available blood sugar or, with competitive sport, an adrenal surge can lead to a see-saw effect, resulting again in low blood sugar.

Sportspeople are therefore often advised to eat fruit or have drinks that will sustain the blood sugar, such as bananas. With endurance sports, such as marathons, a high carbohydrate preparation diet is essential several days before the event. This is recommended to ensure that adequate liver and muscle stores of glycogen are available for conversion into blood glucose, as and when required during the race.

THE STRESS FACTOR MIGRAINE

As already stated, an inappropriately rapid or severe fall in the blood sugar – for whatever reason – can trigger an adrenal compensation. Adrenalin facilitates the release of stored glucose (known as glycogen and stored in the liver and muscle), thus increasing the blood sugar level into the normal range.

However, stress also causes the body to release adrenalin. This mechanism has been termed the 'flight and fight' response to stress. Unfortunately, unlike the sudden short-term stress experienced by animals in the wild, the stress suffered by people in the twentieth century is often of a chronic daily character. The resulting adrenal overactivity and high levels of blood sugar can produce a similar effect to a high sugar diet, with all its far-reaching consequences. In the context of migraine cause, the normal sugar-insulin balance can be gradually altered in favour of low blood sugar. Excessive stress can also cause adrenal exhaustion or hypo-adrenalism – which can again lead to low levels of blood sugar.

THE SUGAR TRIGGER

Although we know that chocolate can cause migraine (chiefly because it contains the vaso-active amine phenylethylamine), many other sugar-rich foods and drinks can also lead to migraine. The rebound effect, so characteristic of the blood changes in migraine, is well demonstrated with a high sugar diet. This type of diet 'trains' the body to produce too much insulin (hyper-insulinism) in response to the sugar, and this creates the paradox of high sugar ingestion resulting in low blood sugar.

HOW DOES HYPOGLYCAEMIA CAUSE MIGRAINE?

It seems useful at this point to discuss just why a drop in our blood sugar can lead to a severe debilitating migraine.

Although the human body utilizes fats and sugars as fuel, glucose is virtually the only fuel required by the brain and nervous system. When glucose is in short supply, the nervous tissue takes priority over the other tissues. It is known that the total supply of glucose to the brain would be exhausted in 10 to 15 minutes, if automatic compensatory reactions failed to work fol-lowing a sudden fall in the blood sugar. Whatever the cause of low blood sugar, be it stress-induced or food-induced, migraine can be the result. This mechanism, whereby a drop in the blood sugar leads to migraine, needs to be explained.

It is generally accepted that over 100 different types of headaches have been identified, and migraine falls under the classification of a vascular headache. This is a headache caused by changes in the blood circulation system.

When the blood sugar in the brain falls below a certain concentration, there occurs an automatic local increase in the blood volume. As I have explained, the body will not tolerate the brain's glucose supply falling below a certain level. This means that reduced blood quality (i.e. low glucose) is compensated for by increased blood quantity. Studies have confirmed that there occurs a marked increase in the blood flow to the brain after insulin-induced low blood sugar. Unfortunately, this increase to the local brain blood supply can lead to a heightening sensitivity of the brain tissue, caused by the expanding or stretching of the blood vessels passing through the brain.

This explains the throbbing pain so characteristic of vascular (circulatory) headaches, and the extreme sensitivity and pain that can occur in migraine over a small localized area (e.g. above one eye). In addition to the localized, often pounding, headache so typical of migraine, the major nerves in the area can be disturbed. These include the cranial nerves which supply the liver, eyes, ears, face, digestive system and other areas. Irritation of these nerves can give rise to the many symptoms so common to the migraine syndrome, including nausea, photophobia and dizziness.

MIGRAINE—TRIGGERS OR CAUSE?

It has been established that there are many migraine triggers, and it is assumed that these triggers cause migraine. You may hear such comments as 'Cheese causes my migraine' or 'Red wine gives me migraine'. I believe that, for a great number of migraine sufferers, a major cause of their problem is low blood sugar. This creates a background tendency to migraine, for reasons already explained. The trigger factors in many cases worsen the problem or act as the 'final straw'.

Significantly, when migraine patients are treated successfully for their low blood sugar, they often discover that they can eat their culprit foods with impunity and that many of their previous triggers no longer cause migraine.

It is usual to define these food triggers as food allergies. I do feel, however, that perhaps many of the suspect foods should be redefined as food intolerances. Chapter 2 looks more closely at migraine triggers and their relationship with existing low blood sugar conditions. Although identifying – and perhaps initially avoiding food triggers – seems a sensible first step in migraine treatment, I do feel that to diagnose and treat any existing low blood sugar should take priority.

It is appropriate to quote a recent book on migraine (1994) by Dr Mike Smith who writes, 'I believe that we shall hear a lot more about the effects of low blood sugar (hypoglycaemia) before too long ...'. Various foods may trigger a migraine attack, but low blood sugar is frequently the *real* cause. Very occasionally, however, the low blood sugar is secondary to a food allergy. The low blood sugar can only then be relieved when the food allergies are identified and removed.

CHAPTER FIVE

The Low Blood Sugar Diet

When treating low blood sugar and migraine there are two problems that I am frequently asked to explain. Patients who are diagnosed as suffering from low blood sugar are confused when advised to avoid sugar. It seems to them quite logical to eat more of any substance that they are told they lack (i.e. glucose). This rule usually applies, after all, to deficiencies of other nutrients such as vitamins and minerals. There is also concern that their diet, prescribed for treating low blood sugar is almost identical to the diet prescribed for *high* blood sugar (diabetes). Yet by definition the two conditions are virtually opposites.

The answer to this mystery lies in the fact that while the two conditions are opposite in terms of blood chemistry and insulin use, the causes of both are very similar. In fact, late-onset diabetes often succeeds low blood sugar, and both conditions are partly caused by the modern diet which tends to be high in sugar and refined sugar-rich foods.

The influence of diet on diabetes is more pronounced

in late-onset diabetes than it is in childhood diabetes, where inheritance plays the dominant role. Many middle-aged diabetics have a previous history of low blood sugar symptoms, including migraine, asthma, obesity and fatigue. Excessive sugar can lead to excessive insulin and low blood sugar. This leads to pancreatic exhaustion, and the low insulin output of the diabetic. In simple terms – overwork followed by exhaustion and underwork. This scenario is very common, and when it occurs any low blood sugar symptoms (migraine, asthma etc.), tend to improve as the low blood sugar recedes and the 'protective' role of diabetes becomes apparent.

THE IDEAL DIET

If low blood sugar is suspected as a cause of migraine, the ideal diet should follow certain ground rules:

1 Sugar in all forms and sugar-rich foods must be avoided. This is a long list, including brown and white sugar, honey, cakes, biscuits, chocolate etc. Care is needed when reading labels, and look out for 'hidden' sugars, including dextrose, molasses, sucrose etc.
2 Wholegrain, unrefined carbohydrates are always to be preferred to the refined variety. For example:
   – 100 per cent wholemeal bread in place of white bread
   – brown rice rather than white rice
   – wholegrain pasta rather than the refined variety.

3 There should be at least four meals daily, with, if possible, a maximum time of three hours between meals. Between-meal snacks can fill in any longer gaps.

4 Breakfast should be eaten as early as possible and the last meal (or supper) as late as possible.

5 Every meal must have a fat or protein component. This will delay absorption of any carbohydrates and also delay the subsequent insulin response.

The Glycaemic Index in Appendix B on page 79 shows the absorption rate of the major foods. The lower the index number, the better the food for this type of diet. This index, first used in the 1970s, gives glucose an arbitrary index of 100, other examples being white bread – 95, wholemeal bread – 50, wholewheat pasta – 30, and green vegetables less than 15.

Remember, the slower the absorption, the less likelihood of sudden swings in the blood sugar, with subsequent sugar and food craving. Following a diet based on correct use of the glycaemic index for food selection can also help those wishing to lose weight.

6 Substances that are known to increase the blood sugar also need to be avoided. These include caffeine, alcohol and tobacco.

Meal Frequency and Night Fasting

A common theme in the many diets recommended for treating low blood sugar is the emphasis on meal frequency and the avoidance of a long night fast. Small regular meals or snacks, consisting of whole complex carbohydrates with protein or fat, help to stabilize the blood sugar, avoiding sudden rises and falls.

The advice to patients to avoid a prolonged night fast often leads to the question, 'If fasting lowers the blood sugar, why do patients in health hydros feel so good on three to five-day fruit juice fasts?' In fact, such patients usually feel pretty awful for the initial 48 hours of the fast, and their blood sugar does indeed fall! However, prolonging a fast does not cause a severe and progressive lowering of the blood sugar. The body utilizes fat and protein reserves to stabilize the blood sugar level. This is a process known as *endogenous catabolism*. With this in mind, researchers have observed that patients who are dying of cancer and unable to eat for lengthy periods have maintained normal blood sugar levels. However, this compensation does not take place until a person has fasted for at least 48 hours.

The Low Blood Sugar Diet and The Food Combining Diet

Many migraine sufferers claim benefits from following the food combining (Hay) diet. This diet, with its emphasis on the correct combining of food groups and a minimum of four hours between meals, is of great value in treating a host of health problems. However, if it is suspected that low blood sugar is a major trigger component in one's migraine, the food combining diet may not be appropriate.

For the food combining diet to work, fats and proteins should not be eaten at the same meal as carbohydrates. When treating low blood sugar, the fat or protein serves to delay absorption, and reduces the tendency for sudden swings to occur in the blood sugar. The frequent snacks that are required in the initial weeks of treatment contrast with the four-hour rule in the food combining diet. This type of programme is therefore not ideal for treating migraine brought on by low blood sugar. However, if low blood sugar is not a suspected cause then the food combining diet is well worth considering.

It is a question of priorities, and for the majority of migraine sufferers the primary need is to identify and treat the various food triggers.

The Diet for Migraine

So what is the ideal diet for migraine caused chiefly by low blood sugar?

Many of the doctors and nutritionists, who write about and treat low blood sugar problems, advocate their own special diet for this problem. The diets vary according to their fat, protein, and carbohydrate content, although the meal frequency and other 'ground rules' are very similar. (For a detailed analysis of the various types of diets read my book *Low Blood Sugar* in the Thorsons Health Series – see *Recommended Reading*.)

It is sufficient here to outline the basic diet that I prescribe for migraine sufferers with a proven or suspected tendency to low blood sugar, and where no specific food triggers have been identified.

DIET FOR LOW BLOOD SUGAR

- *On rising*
  1 piece of fresh fruit or 4oz (100g) fresh fruit juice.
- *Breakfast*
  1 piece of fresh fruit or 4oz (100g) fresh fruit juice.
  Selection from the following:

  Egg dish (scrambled, boiled or poached).
  Small omelette (plain cheese or mushroom etc.).
  Bacon or sugar-free ham.
  Grilled or steamed fish.
  On toast – cheese, pâté or sardines etc., with sugar-free spread, or sugar-free baked beans.
  Cereal – sugar-free muesli or wholegrain sugar-free cereal with cow's milk or yogurt.
  Yogurt – with or without fruit (natural live sugar-free yogurt is preferred).
  Note Use only 100 per cent stoneground bread.
  To drink: decaffeinated coffee or tea, fresh fruit juice or mineral water.
- *2 hours after breakfast*
  1 piece of fruit or 4oz (100g) fresh fruit juice or a natural yogurt.
- *Lunch*
  Meat, fish, egg or cheese dish with salad or vegetables. With wholemeal bread, wholegrain pasta, brown rice or jacket potato.
  Or as breakfast.
  Dessert: cheese, yogurt or fresh fruit.

To drink: mineral water, fruit juice, or sugar-free decaffeinated beverage.

- *2 hours after lunch:* (and every two hours until dinner) 1 piece of fruit or 4oz (100g) fresh fruit juice.
- *Dinner*

  Soup if desired.

  Portion of meat, fowl or chicken, with vegetables or salad. Include wholegrain pasta, brown rice or jacket potato.

  Dessert: cheese, yogurt or fresh or baked fruit. Beverage if desired.

- *2 hours after dinner (and every two hours until supper)*

  1 piece of fruit or 4oz (100g) fresh fruit juice or milk or yogurt, or small handful of unsalted nuts.

- *Supper (as late as possible)*

  Ryvita or wholemeal bread with cheese, ham, pâté or cold meat with beverage.

Notes: Many sugar-free products are now available. These include sugar-free cereals and muesli, and sugar-free tinned fruit and juices. Diabetic products are best avoided unless sweetened with fructose. Pickles, sauces (unless homemade) and salt should all be avoided. Use low-fat products wherever possible and salt-free butter. The lunch and dinner can be reversed.

Many diets recommended for treating low blood sugar insist on the strict avoidance of carbohydrates (i.e. bread, cereal, rice, pasta and potatoes). I do feel, however, that the complex carbohydrates that have low numbers in the Glycaemic Index (see Appendix B) can be allowed on the diet. To ban all such foods reduces meal variety and food selection, encourages a high fat content in the meals, and, perhaps most important, offers very little fibre in food. I have known patients who have followed the American high-fat (Ketogenic), low-starch diet to develop stubborn constipation and weight increase. Such a diet has also been criticized as a potential cause of heart problems.

The Vegetarian Diet for Low Blood Sugar

Many people are turning to meat-free diets. Although plant proteins are just as valuable as animal proteins, the amino acids (protein components) in fish, fowl and meat are utilized by our digestive systems more easily and efficiently than the protein in plants. It is therefore essential to have plenty of variety in the plant proteins eaten, and a knowledge of vegetarian cooking is an advantage.

- *On rising*
  1 piece of fresh fruit of 4oz (100g) fresh fruit juice.
- *Breakfast*
  1 piece of fresh fruit or 4oz (100g) fresh fruit juice.
  Selection from the following:
  Egg dish (scrambled, poached or boiled).
  Small omelette (plain, cheese or mushroom etc.)
  On toast – cheese, sugar-free baked beans, sugar-free spread or vegetarian pâté.
  Cereal – sugar-free muesli, or wholegrain sugar-free cereal with milk or yogurt.
  Yogurt – with or without fruit (natural live, sugar-free yogurt is preferred).

Note: Use only 100 per cent stoneground wholemeal bread.

To drink: decaffeinated coffee or tea, fresh fruit juice or mineral water.

- *2 hours after breakfast*

    1 piece of fresh fruit or 4oz (100g) fresh fruit juice, or a natural yogurt.

- *Lunch*

    As breakfast, or salad with cheese, eggs, or vegetarian savoury. Ideal dressings include vinegar, lemon juice or sugar-free mayonnaise.

    Wholemeal bread or jacket potato or wholegrain pasta dish.

    To drink: decaffeinated coffee or tea, fruit juice or mineral water.

- *2 hours after lunch (and every two hours until dinner)*

    1 piece of fruit or 4oz (100g) fresh fruit juice.

- *Dinner*

    Soup if desired.

    Mixed vegetables or salad with selection as follows: vegetarian savoury, egg or cheese dish, stuffed peppers, tomatoes or aubergines, savoury rice, wholegrain pasta, lentil savoury, soya dish, etc.

    Dessert: cheese, yogurt, fresh or baked fruit.

    To drink: fresh fruit juice or mineral water.

- *2 hours after dinner (and every two hours up to supper)*

    1 piece of fruit or 4oz (100g) fresh fruit juice or milk, or yogurt, or small handful of unsalted nuts.

- *Supper (as late as possible)*

    Ryvita or wholemeal bread with cheese or vegetarian pâté, with beverage if required or milk.

Notes: Many sugar-free products are now available. These include sugar-free cereals and muesli, and sugar-free tinned fruit and juices. Diabetic products are best avoided unless sweetened with fructose. Pickles, sauces (unless homemade) and salt should all be avoided. Use low-fat products wherever possible and salt-free butter. The lunch and dinner can be reversed.

Vegan Diet for Low Blood Sugar

This is perhaps the most challenging and difficult diet to design and follow. The avoidance of all animal products, including milk, cheese and eggs, does reduce the menu options. However, I outline below the standard diet prescribed for vegans. The book by Paavo Airola, *Hypoglycaemia, a Better Approach* (see *Recommended Reading*), offers a particularly effective treatment programme for vegans and vegetarians.

- *On rising*
  1 piece of fruit or 4oz (100g) fresh fruit juice.
- *Breakfast*
  1 piece of fruit of 4oz (100g) fresh fruit juice.
  On toast – vegan cheese, mushrooms, sugar-free baked beans, vegan pâté (use olive oil or other vegetable spread).
  Cereal – wholegrain sugar-free cereal or muesli with soya milk (can be diluted with fruit juice to taste).
  To drink: decaffeinated coffee or beverage or fruit juice or mineral water.

- *2 hours after breakfast*

  1 piece of fresh fruit, soya milk or 4oz fruit juice (100g).

- *Lunch*

  As breakfast, or salad with vegan cheese or vegan savoury (ideal dressings include cider vinegar, lemon juice or olive oil-based dressing), nuts and fruit.

  Wholemeal bread, jacket potato or wholegrain pasta dish.

  To drink: decaffeinated coffee or tea, soya milk or fruit juice or mineral water.

- *2 hours after lunch (and every two hours until dinner)*

  1 piece of fruit or 4oz (100g) fresh fruit juice.

- *Dinner*

  Soup or piece of fruit

  Mixed vegetables or salad with selection of the following: vegan savoury, stuffed peppers, tomatoes or aubergines, lentil or soya savoury, vegan cheese, vegetable pie or casserole, wholegrain pasta or rice, jacket potato or wholemeal bread.

  Dessert: vegan cheese, nuts, fruit (fresh or baked).

  To drink: soya milk, fruit juice, beverage or mineral water.

- *2 hours after dinner (and every two hours up to supper)*

  1 piece of fruit or 4oz (100g) fresh fruit juice or soya milk, or small handful of unsalted nuts.

- *Supper*

  Ryvita or wholemeal bread with vegan pâté or vegan cheese, with beverage or soya milk if required.

Notes: There are many vegan products now available; olive oil spread makes a good butter substitute. Several books listed in *Recommended Reading* provide vegan, sugar-free recipes (including the book co-written with my wife *Recipes for Health: Low Blood Sugar* by Thorsons).

The Low Blood Sugar Diet – Duration and Progress

If low blood sugar is the main cause of your migraines, these diets should reduce the incidence and severity of your symptoms within six to eight weeks.

This assumes that any known food triggers are avoided and your migraines occur on a regular and predictable basis. If your migraines only occur three or four times annually, any symptom relief will be very difficult to assess. It must also be said that migraines which only develop three or four times each year are very rarely linked to any food triggers (unless, of course, known triggers are inadvertently eaten).

CHAPTER SIX

The Adrenal Link

For the greater part of the twentieth century, doctors and nutritionists have tested for, demonstrated and treated the connection between food and migraine. One question, however, has never been fully answered. Why are some people sensitive to certain foods and yet the majority are not?

Those who suffer migraine symptoms, and show an allergic response to specific foods, very often show similar symptoms and personality patterns. These characteristics are summarized below as follows. Perhaps you fit this model?

THE ALLERGIC PERSONALITY

Those who are subject to allergies are often hardworking perfectionists, who find it very difficult to relax. They are usually anxious, irritable and easily fatigued. Their conversion of food to energy is not very efficient. They tend to have a poor body thermostat, and do not tolerate extreme heat or cold. Insomnia and low blood pressure are common symptoms, coupled with poor stress-handling. Ease of bruising, coldness of hands and feet, and muscular cramps are commonplace. Allergy sufferers are not good in the morning, often waking with dark shadows around their eyes and feeling very sluggish (mentally and physically). All these symptoms tend to improve by the afternoon. Exercise is not favoured and, although they frequently crave sugar, their weight is usually normal. Is this a fair description of your symptoms?

Adrenal problems and allergies

If we recognize the concept of a typical allergy type, whether applied to migraine, asthma or skin conditions etc., it follows that there is probably a common cause to allergic symptoms and personalities. I believe that there *is* a common component to allergies and low blood sugar problems, this being the role of the adrenal glands. These paired glands lie over each kidney and produce a range of vital hormones that influence many aspects of our metabolism. Dr Tintera, an internationally recognized specialist in endocrine treatment, stated in 1956 that, 'Migraine is a symptom of glandular disorder'.

In America the term 'nervous breakdown' is rarely used. The expression *adrenal exhaustion* is preferred and considered more appropriate. 'Exhaustion' suggest a reversible, functional condition and not a disease or damage (disease of the adrenal glands is termed

Addison's disease). Some specialists prefer to use the term sub-clinical Addison's to define inefficient adrenal glands. The same experts point to weak or overworked adrenal glands as being the chief cause of many illnesses. The outer part of the adrenal gland (the cortex) produces the corticosteroids (cortisone and cortisol) and sex hormones. The corticosteroids are prescribed to treat cancers, allergies and all types of inflammation. In addition they are used to suppress immune responses and for hormone replacement therapy. The adrenal centre (medulla) produces adrenalin and noradrenalin. These hormones prepare to body to handle stress, and to raise the blood sugar.

This helps us to understand the role that the adrenal glands play in causing such apparently diverse health problems as fatigue, anxiety, depression, joint and muscle pain, female hormone conditions, low blood sugar and allergies.

ADRENAL EXHAUSTION

When the adrenal glands become exhausted and inefficient, it was thought in the early days of hormone research that cortisone offered a safe answer. Its near miraculous effect on joint pain, allergies, skin rashes, bowel problems and general well-being, tended to confirm the initial high hopes. Unfortunately, cortisone also causes side effects, which can include hyperglycaemia (raised blood sugar), high blood-pressure, eye damage and disease, impotence, mood changes, moon face (water and fat imbalance), kidney stones, poor wound healing, muscle weakness, osteoporosis and general chemical imbalances throughout the body.

In addition to these effects it was found, in common with many other hormone treatments, that to prescribe cortisone for an already weakened adrenal system tended to create a long-term reliance on the drug. This led to a resulting reduction in the patient's own cortisone production. In fact, the use of hormones in therapy often has the effect of training our own glands to be less efficient. A more logical and less harmful approach to adrenal exhaustion, or *hypoadrenalism*, is called for. This involves the three-pronged programme, as outlined below.

1 Stress adjustment

This is perhaps the most difficult part of the programme: to recognize and to come to terms with the causes of our stress, and perhaps to change the attitudes or habits of a lifetime, is never easy. We may need to learn how to control our responses to stress, and to understand the physical and mental damage that can be caused by stress. Sometimes a reappraisal of family and work pressures is a good starting point. Counselling, relaxation techniques, hypnotherapy, yoga and biofeedback are all valuable aids to achieve a new state of relaxation.

It is always worth remembering that there occurs a chemical activity in the brain every time we think. The efficient handling of stress is not simply a matter of willpower or personal strength of character. The stress management and treatment depends ultimately on our adrenal glands, and their effective and appropriate response to the stress.

2 Correct diet

The ideal diet for hypoadrenalism is identical to the diet that is recommended for the treatment of low blood sugar (see Chapter 5.) Low blood sugar will trigger adrenal activity, so a diet aimed at stabilizing any swings in the level of sugar in the blood will indirectly support the adrenals. This diet will impose minimum strain on a weak or exhausted adrenal system, and in doing so lead to a better level of health and vitality. As we know, a poorly functioning adrenal system can cause food sensitivity and low blood sugar. It may be that the chief difference between stressed, allergic individuals and the healthier majority lies in their adrenal health and efficiency.

It should be remembered that the adrenal glands are at the centre of our bodies' 'defence administration'. Our chemistry does not welcome the invasion of foreign substances, whether they are viruses, poisons or bacteria. It is the adrenal hormones which provide the necessary defence and immune efficiency. If these vital glands are not working correctly then we are open to widespread chemical imbalance.

3 Adrenal support

In addition to improved stress awareness and handling, and correct eating, there are specific nutritional supplements that can support an exhausted adrenal system. These include tissue concentrates (glandulars), that are prescribed to enhance the function of a specific gland. They come from a healthy bovine source of South American cattle.

Vitamins are also of value, in particular the whole vitamin B family, especially vitamin B$_5$, vitamin C and vitamin E. The following herbals are also used in adrenal formulae: ginseng, liquorice, wild yam, gota kola and valerian. The minerals magnesium, chromium, zinc and manganese are also often included for adrenal support.

CHAPTER SEVEN

Diets to Help Migraine

Readers will by now appreciate that no single diet is suitable to treat every type of migraine. To design a diet that avoids the vaso-active amines in food, identifies and eliminates potential allergy triggers and also treats any low blood sugar tendency is – to say the least – very difficult.

The answer to every migraine sufferer's question, 'So what is my ideal diet?' needs to be carefully considered. A logical step-by-step process of detection is essential in order to arrive at an enjoyable and effective diet.

STEP 1

The first step deals with the smallest group of triggers – the vaso-active amines. The foods and drinks which contain the amines are discussed in Chapter 1. These are well-known, common triggers, and many migraineurs know only too well the effect that they have on their symptoms. Avoidance is relatively simple and, fortunately, the list does not contain any indispensable foods or drinks that cannot be substituted. Even cheese, a common trigger, can often be safely replaced by vegetarian cheese or the soft goats' milk or sheep's milk variety. Although citrus fruits and juices are a common and valuable source of Vitamin C, there are many alternative fruits available to replace them. Only potatoes are difficult to substitute but the total amount of vaso-active amines (tyramine) in potatoes is minimal, and for this reason potatoes alone very rarely act as migraine triggers.

A sensible first step would be to avoid completely the whole vaso-active amine group and then assess progress over a four to six week period. This assumes that you would normally experience migraine symptoms within this time period. Potatoes could be gradually re-introduced if symptom-relief is achieved, and any reaction noted. If a migraine is *not* triggered, it can be assumed that potatoes are not one of the food culprits.

Fortunately this group does not include foods that belong to large families, nor are they often 'hidden' in processed or prepared mixes and recipes. They are usually very easy to identify in our diet and therefore easy to avoid.

A further refinement in understanding the effect of this group of triggers is to reintroduce the foods and drinks into your diet one at a time, on the basis of eating one item every five to seven days. Again, this is assuming that the initial avoidance of the whole group has led to symptom relief.

You may discover in this way that although cheese and red wine trigger symptoms, citrus fruits and chocolate do not. If, however, complete symptom-relief is only achieved by avoiding *all* the vaso-active amine-rich foods and drinks, any future treatment would consist of simply avoiding the whole group and introducing suitable alternatives into your diet. For further details of food substitutes, see Appendix C, page 82.

Should Step 1 prove ineffective and your migraines persist, it would be fair to assume that other factors are triggering your symptoms. With this is mind, the next step is to look at the low blood sugar connection. Because identifying and treating food allergy triggers is both complex and time consuming, it seems sensible to leave the allergy triggers to the final step.

Step 2

By now you will have realized that I believe that functional hypoglycaemia (low blood sugar) is a common migraine trigger. However, although it can be interesting and reassuring to be given a diagnosis of low blood sugar following an extended glucose tolerance test, it may not be much help when treating migraine. Many people with low blood sugar do *not* suffer migraine, so it may be misleading to conclude that such a diagnosis is the sole cause of your migraine.

A little detective work is needed here to link your migraine symptoms to low blood sugar situations. In this way a logical cause and effect pattern can be identified. Although this subject is covered in detail in Chapter 2, a few simple examples will refresh your memory.

Low Blood Sugar Triggers – the clues

1 The symptoms usually start in the early hours, usually 3 to 4 a.m.
2 The symptoms may only occur at weekends after a lie-in or a late breakfast.
3 The symptoms seem to develop shortly after stress, such as a family argument, work pressures etc.
4 The symptoms usually develop late afternoon if lunch is missed, or just before lunch if breakfast is missed.
5 The symptoms only occur pre-menstrually.
6 The symptoms occur mainly after sport or exercise.

The common theme to these migraine patterns is low blood sugar, which may fall too quickly, or to an unacceptably low level, thus triggering symptoms.

If you have not obtained any symptom-relief after following the diet outlined in Step 1, but you believe that there may be a low blood sugar trigger, you should now return to Chapter 6 and follow the recommended diet.

To assess its value, you should follow the low blood sugar diet for six to eight weeks, as the symptoms should begin to improve within this time if changes in the blood sugar are causing your migraine. Obviously, if there is no symptom-relief, it is very unlikely that a tendency to low blood sugar is the main trigger component in your migraine. As with the vaso-active amine triggers, this assumption is only valid if you would normally and predictably suffer migraine symptoms on a regular basis (i.e. at least one attack per month).

Step 3

The food allergy diet for treating migraines is by defini-tion a diet that exclude *known* food allergies. The clue to designing and successfully following such a diet is the word *known*. It is obviously essential to identify the foods that trigger your migraines.

The subject of food allergy testing is discussed in detail in Chapter 5. There are many different proce-dures for allergy testing, ranging from blood tests to muscle testing and pulse measurement. However, this book is essentially a guide to self-treatment along dietary lines, and it may be helpful to look again at the methods used to identify your own food allergies.

Elimination – Provocation Testing

Designing a limited or rare food diet is a logical first step in identifying food allergies. The aim of this type of diet is to exclude all the common migraine-causing foods in order to achieve symptom relief. If the symptoms are *not* improved then it is unlikely that food allergies play a part in causing your migraine. You are advised to select foods that are rarely or never eaten in your routine diet. In this way you will ensure that foods which usually trigger your symptoms will not be inad-vertently included in the diet.

After the initial period (usually three to four weeks) on a limited food diet which (hopefully) leads to symp-tom relief, the next stage is to introduce common foods on a challenge basis. The normal daily amounts of each of the excluded foods are introduced at least twice daily for three consecutive days and, if symptoms are provoked, these foods are not included in the diet. If *no* symptoms develop, then the safe foods are systematically added to the diet until the diet is nutritionally balanced and quite acceptable to the tester (from social and economic viewpoints). Allergic responses can be very rapid or very slow, and migraine symptoms usually develop from one to 48 hours after eating a sensitive food. So you should allow at least three days after eating a food to assess its effect. If no symptoms arise within this time, then the food is safe for you to eat. This means that a new food can be introduced and tested every six to seven days.

Elimination Diet – Recommended Schedule of Foods

This diet is based on the assumption that rarely eaten foods are unlikely to cause symptoms. If you normally eat any of these foods more than once a week they should not be in your diet. They are as follows:

- *Proteins*
  Lamb, turkey, duck, goose, rabbit, guinea fowl, venison, pheasant and any fish (not smoked or shellfish).
- *Vegetables*
  Celeriac, celery, asparagus, mange-tout, avocado, lettuce, cress, watercress, spinach.

- *Carbohydrates*
  Rice, buckwheat, yams, pumpkin, sago, turnips, parsnips, tapioca, millet.
- *Fruit*
  Pears, blackcurrants, redcurrants, gooseberries, kiwi fruit, lychees, mangoes, bananas, pomegranate, passion-fruit.
- *Fats and Oils*
  Any single source, first pressed oil, avoiding animal fat.
- *Snacks*
  Sunflower seeds, pine nuts, cashew nuts, chestnuts, brazil nuts.
- *Drinks*
  Only glass-bottled mineral water.

Note: If the initial three to four week exclusion diet based on a selection from this list does not provide symptom-relief, it would be advisable to follow a diet based on a different selection of rare foods, again for three to four weeks.

Points to Note

1 You may feel worse for a few days after stopping a food. These withdrawal symptoms are seen as a good sign, and symptom-relief is usually obtained after six to seven days.
2 When a reaction to a food occurs, stop eating the food. The symptoms produced by an allergic response can be reduced by taking 2 teaspoons of bicarbonate of soda and 1 teaspoon of potassium bicarbonate, in a

glass of warm water. Do not introduce any further foods until the symptoms have completely ceased.

3 If a reintroduced food causes symptoms, the pulse test (see page 21), is a useful confirmation of sensitivity.

4 Keep a diary of foods eaten, reactions to foods and suspected foods over at least the initial reintroduction phase.

5 Buy good quality, fresh unprocessed food. This particularly applies to meats. Wash fruit and vegetables thoroughly before eating.

6 Avoid anything *not* in your food lists, in particular condiments, sauces, pickles etc.

7 The taking of all supplements, herbs, vitamins, and *unnecessary* drugs should be discontinued with the onset of the elimination diet.

Reintroduction Diet – Recommended Schedule

The choice of foods to be tested on a basis of systematic reintroduction will vary according to individual taste. However, there are some common foods that should be tested initially, which are as follows: milk, cheese, yeast extract (Marmite), citrus fruits (oranges and lemons), eggs, chicken, beef, rice, wheat and other cereals, tea, coffee, wine (red and white), potatoes.

It would be advisable to plan your strategy by listing your own favourite foods, and ensuring that they are included in your reintroduction programme of suspected foods to be tested. But it is important that you only test one food at a time. Start on day one with a portion of the food at two meals. If no reaction occurs, repeat the next day, and if no reaction again repeat for the third day. If there are no reactions, then the food can be added to your menu and considered non-sensitive. Is it essential to test the foods in a pure form without added ingredients, for example test wheat as a cereal with water or fruit juice and *not* as bread.

Other examples of this are:

– To test oats, test as porridge with water.
– To test rye, test as pure rye crispbread.
– To test barley, test as pearl barley and water.
– To test maize (corn), test as sweetcorn.

Prolonged avoidance of a food that you know can cause migraine symptoms can lead in time to a loss of sensitivity to the food, i.e. it becomes 'acceptable' again. Many people may take years to lose 'intolerance' – in others six to eight weeks is sufficient. It is therefore a wise move to test for major suspect foods within the initial eight week period. Furthermore, the most likely food culprit should be tested first. If after eight weeks there are some foods still to test you could reintroduce them on the basis of two to three foods each day for a week and observe any symptoms. If no symptoms develop they can be considered safe.

If a reaction does occur, avoid them all for seven days and go back to Stage 1, i.e. reintroducing one food at a time. This procedure will take approximately three months, but your final diet should be acceptable to you and keep you symptom-free. Most migraine sufferers consider that three months of special diets is a small price to pay for eventual symptom relief.

If you find that some of the foods that cause your symptoms are amongst your favourites, you could retest. However this must be after a six-month period. If you are still intolerant of the food you could test again in another six months. If after such time you are no longer sensitive, the food could then be eaten on a four to five day rotation basis. If you have at one time been very sensitive to a food, it is never advisable to reintroduce it on a daily basis.

See also Appendix C on page 82 for details of food substitutes.

Multiple or Mixed Food Triggers

There is evidence that some migraine sufferers are sensitive to 20 or more different foods. If this is suspected, or the elimination–reintroduction form of self-testing becomes too protracted or offers no relief, then perhaps professional allergy testing would be appropriate.

Lack of symptom improvement may be due to other health problems in addition to food allergies. If the migraines persist, the following should be considered in this context.

- candidiasis (*Candida Albicans*)
- intestinal parasites
- nutritional deficiencies
- lactobacillus and bifidobacteria deficiencies
- deficiency of digestive enzymes

- malabsorption or 'leaky gut' syndrome
- achlorhydria (deficiency of gastric hydrochloric acid)
- virus infections
- psychosomatic disorders
- structural causes of headaches, e.g. jaw or neck mis-alignments
- chemical sensitivities, for example from various fumes, sprays, smokes, vapours, solvents, food additives, pollutants in drinking water, drug side-effects, pesticide residues in food and drink, and perfumes.
- serious neurological disease or damage (e.g. brain tumour)
- electro-magnetic radiations, for example from VDUs, word processors etc.
- side-effects of HRT or the contraceptive pill
- chronic fatigue states
- hypothyroidism
- disorders of the liver or pancreas

NUTRITIONAL SUPPLEMENTS AND MIGRAINE

Many vitamins, minerals and nutritional substances have proven to be of value in treating migraine.

The supplements commonly prescribed for the different types of migraines are listed below.

- *To improve circulation and blood flow*
  Vitamin E
  Niacin (Vitamin B$_3$)

Vitamin B complex
Calcium
Bioflavonoids (Quercetin, Pynogenal and Rutin etc.)
Vitamin C
Ginger and Feverfew
Evening Primrose Oil
Vitamin B_{12}.

- *Allergy Headaches*
Calcium
Beta carotene
Vitamin B_5 (pantothenic acid).
Vitamin C
Bioflavonoids (Quercetin, Pynogenal and Rutin etc.)
Bromelain.
- *Menstrual headaches*
Vitamin B_6
Feverfew
Ovarian glandular products
Essential fatty acids (Evening Primrose Oil, Black-currant Seed Oil, Linseed Oil etc.)
- *Low blood sugar headaches*
Glucose tolerance factor
Chromium
Magnesium
Vitamin B complex
Glandular pancreatic and adrenal products
Vitamin C
Vitamin B_{12}
- *Stress headaches*
Adrenal glandular products
As *Low blood sugar* listings

Valerian – Skull Cap – Passion Flower.
Vitamin B complex
Sodium chloride (salt).

- *General*

Potassium chloride (soluble) is of value in non-stress headaches. High-dose vitamin B_{12} is indicated if headaches are chronic with fatigue and/or vomiting. High-dose calcium is useful with Vitamin C to prevent allergy headaches. This combination should be taken 30 minutes before and immediately after each meal.

OTHER THERAPIES

Acupuncture

I find this ancient therapy of particular value in treating migraine when there is a digestive or liver component, i.e. vomiting and fatigue. It can be particularly helpful when coupled with high dosage intramuscular vitamin B_{12} injections.

Osteopathy and chiropractic

Many migraines are relieved, sometimes permanently, by correcting misalignments in the neck vertebrae. This applies in particular to those sufferers who have experienced whiplash injuries (sustained in road traffic accidents or even riding dodgem cars in fairgrounds). It is usually advisable to obtain X-rays prior to treatment if trauma is in your history. Special remedial pillow-use may be needed.

Cranial osteopathy

This specialized form of osteopathic treatment is considered by many practitioners to have a unique value in the treatment of migraine and other types of headaches.

CONCLUSION

Self-help for most health problems is worthwhile if the diagnosis is correct and the cause identified. However it should be remembered that severe headaches may not be migraine headaches but something much more serious. A self-diagnosis or a wrong diagnosis may allow time for the problem to become untreatable.

Conditions that may mimic migraine symptoms include the following:

temporal arteritis
brain tumour
glaucoma
intra cerebral haemorrhage (stroke)
high blood-pressure
iron deficient anaemia
acute sinusitis
encephalitis
dental abscess
meningitis

trigeminal neuralgia
hormonal problems (thyroid, pituitary, ovaries, etc.)

If your symptoms are unusual, without an obvious cause or very severe, you should *always* seek professional help.

There are many excellent books written on every aspect of migraine diagnosis and treatment. Some of these are listed under *Recommended Reading* on page 87. Details of supplement dosages and herbal remedies should be obtained from an appropriate professional practitioner. The dosage recommended on containers is usually a guide to maintenance dosage. Individual requirements can vary with different health problems.

Appendix A: Food Families

PLANTS

Banana Family *(Musaceae)*
Banana, plantain, arrowroot.
Bean and Pea Family *(Leguminoseae)*
All types of peas and beans including soya, lentils, peanut, liquorice, kidney beans, haricot beans, green peas, mung beans and alfalfa etc.
Buckwheat Family *(Polygoaceae)*
Buckwheat, rhubarb, garden sorrel.
Cabbage or Mustard Family *(Cruciferae)*
Broccoli, Brussels sprouts, cabbage, cauliflower, Chinese leaves, horseradish, kale, swede, turnip, kohlrabi, cress and watercress, spring greens, rape.
Carrot or Parsley Family *(Umbelliferae)*
Carrot, celery, celeriac, fennel, parsnip, aniseed, parsley, coriander, dill, cumin, caraway, chervil, lovage and sweet cicely.
Cashew Family *(Anacardiaceae)*
Cashew, pistachio, mango.

Citrus or Rue Family *(Rutaceae)*
Lemon, orange, grapefruit, lime, tangerine, clementine and kumquat.

Cucumber or Gourd Family *(Cucurbitaceae)*
Cucumber, melon, marrow, courgette, watermelon, pumpkin, squash and gherkin.

Daisy or Composite Family *(Compositae)*
Lettuce, chicory, artichoke, endive, salsify, safflower, sunflower, dandelion, burdock root and camomile.

Fungi and Moulds
Yeast, mushrooms, cheese mould, truffles and vinegar.

Grape Family *(Vitaceae)*
Grapes, raisins, sultanas, currants, wine, brandy, sherry, wine vinegar, cream of tartar.
(Note Black and redcurrants are in the currant family.)

Grass Family *(Gramineae)*
Wheat, maize (corn), barley, oats, rye, millet, bamboo, sugar cane, rice and sorghum.
(Note Buckwheat is not in this family.)

Sub-Families:

Bambusoideae
Rice and wild rice.
Chloridoideae
Millet.
Panacoideae
Maize (corn), sugar cane and sorghum.
Pooidae
Wheat, barley, rye and oats.

Mint Family *(Labiatae)*
Thyme, sage, catnip, hyssop, lavender, savory, peppermint, mint, oregano, marjoram, basil, rosemary.

Mulberry Family *(Moraceae)*
Figs, hops, mulberry and breadfruit.

Onion or Lily Family *(Liliaceae)*
Onions, leeks, garlic, shallots, asparagus, aloe vera, yucca, sarsaparilla, chives and spring onions.

Palm Family *(Palmaceae)*
Coconut, sago, date.

Potato Family *(Solanaceae)*
Aubergine, potato, tomato, tobacco, pepper (red, green and yellow), paprika, chilli, cayenne.

Rose Family *(Rosaceae)*
This large family sub-divides as follows:

Maloideae (Pomes)
Pear, apple, loquat and quince.

Prunoideae (Stone fruits)
Prune, plum, apricot, greengage, peach, cherry, nectarine, sloe, almond.

Rosoideae (Berries)
Blackberry, dewberry, loganberry, raspberry, strawberry, rosehip.

Spinach or Goosefoot Family *(Chenopodiaceae)*
Spinach, chard, sugar-beet and beetroot.

Walnut Family *(Juglandaceae)*
Walnut, pecans and hickory nuts.

FISH

All bony fish share a protein known as *parvalbumin*. This can cause allergies, which explains why some people are sensitive to *all* types of fish.

Other fish families include:

Molluscs *(Phylum Mollusca)*
Snail, squid, octopus, abalone, clam, mussel, scallop, oyster, winkles, cuttlefish.

Crustaceans *(Phylum Crustacea)*
Prawn, lobster, crab, crayfish, shrimp.

MEAT

Ruminants
Cows, (veal and beef), sheep, (lamb, mutton), goats. Milk and dairy products.

Poultry and Eggs

Duck Family *(Anatidae)*
Duck and goose.

Grouse Sub-family *(Tetraoninae)*
Grouse, turkey, guineafowl.

Pheasant Sub-family *(Phasianinae)*
Chicken, quail, pheasant, partridge.

Pigeon Family *(Columbidae)*
Pigeon, dove, squab (young pigeon).

Snipe Family *(Scolopacidae)*
Woodcock and snipe.

Pig Family *(Suidae)*
Pig, (pork, ham, bacon), wild boar.

Deer Family *(Cervidae)*
Venison.
Rabbit Family *(Leporidae)*
Hare and rabbit.

NOTES

Sensitivity to one member of a food family does not automatically imply sensitivity to the whole family. However, this possibility should be considered when designing a rotation diet. Juices, oils, beverages, seeds, extracts and the products of a particular plant may cause symptoms if the whole plant is an allergen.

Many plants, fish and animals do not belong to a family but are 'one-offs'. For example:
- Plants: pineapple, poppyseed, caper, gooseberry, flaxseed, tea, papaya, olive and many nuts.
- Meat: venison, ostrich, anchovy.

Appendix B:
The Glycaemic Index

SUGARS

Glucose 100
Honey 87
Sucrose 59
Fructose 20

CEREALS

Cornflakes... 80
Wholegrain bread 72
White rice 72
White bread 69
Brown rice 68
Shredded wheat.. 67
Swiss muesli 66
Sweetcorn... 59
All Bran 51
Spaghetti.. 50

Oatmeal cereal	49
Wholewheat spaghetti	42

FRUIT

Raisins	64
Banana	62
Orange juice	46
Apple juice	45
Orange	40
Apple	39

VEGETABLES

Parsnip	97
Carrot	92
Mashed potato	80
Potato	70
Beetroot	64
Frozen peas	51
Peas	33

PULSES

Baked beans	40
Lima beans	36
Kidney beans	29
Lentils	29
Soya beans	15

DAIRY PRODUCTS

VARIOUS

Appendix C:
Substitute Foods
and Drinks

When you are avoiding specific foods and drinks to which you are sensitive, it is very helpful to know what you can safely use as a substitute. For more detailed information, you would be advised to write directly to the York Nutritional Laboratory and request their *Food Sensitivity Guidebook* (cost £4.99, including postage and packing, see address under *Recommended reading*). Another very useful book is Rita Greer's *Wheat, Milk and Egg-free Cooking* (published by Thorsons).

COWS' MILK AND DAIRY PRODUCTS

An allergy to cows' milk does not necessarily include sensitivity to goats' or sheep's milk or their products. It is quite easy nowadays to obtain goats' and sheep's yogurt, cheese and milk from the major food stores.

Soya milk and soya milk products also make good substitutes. Soya milk is available either sweetened or unsweetened, it is more palatable when it is chilled and diluted with 25 to 30 per cent mineral water. Natural flavourings can be added if wished. Rice milk and nut milks are also available. Vegetable or fruit puree can be added to baked food in place of milk, and this improves the texture.

Vegetable oil (preferably mono or polyunsaturated, such as olive or sunflower oil) can replace butter in cooking. Other substitutes for butter include soya or vegan margarine, vegetable spreads and polyunsaturated margarines (although these may contain whey – check the label first). Tomato juice or puree can be used in place of milk in casseroles and meat dishes.

Cheese

An allergy to cheese made from cows' milk may allow you to eat goats' or sheep's milk cheese. This offers a huge range of hard and soft cheeses.

Vegan cheeses which are based on soya products (tofu), may also be purchased from health food stores. Grilled, smoked or marinated tofu may also be acceptable substitutes for cheese.

CHOCOLATE, WINE AND CITRUS FRUITS

Chocolate cannot be replaced by cocoa, unfortunately, because cocoa is used to make chocolate. However, carob can be an acceptable substitute as it has a similar flavour but contains none of the troublesome amines and no caffeine either. Carob powder can be used in cooling and is also available as bars, drops etc. Most health food stores stock it in a variety of different products.

Red wine can be a trigger for some people who may find, however, that rosé and white wines are less likely to bring on a migraine. Drinking plenty of water with wine can help to lessen the effects or, alternatively, non-alcoholic grape juice may be an acceptable substitute.

If citrus fruits are to be excluded from the diet, other vitamin C-rich foods should be substituted, such as leafy green vegetables. Where lemon juice is needed in cooking, vitamin C powder can be used instead. But good quality malt or cider vinegar can be added to sauces and salad dressings instead of lemon juice and it can be a helpful raising agent in cakes when heavier flour than wheat flour is needed.

WHEAT

Wheat is not easy to avoid or to substitute, being so widely used in a range of foods. It is often 'hidden' in soups, sauces, prepared meats (pâtés etc.) and many processed foods. This wheat is often referred to as 'edible starch'.

Remember that wheat belongs to the Grass family, which also includes barley, corn, millet, oats, rice and rye. Substitute flours excluding the above are as listed below. All are equal to *one* cup of wheat flour:

Sago flour	1½ cups
Tapioca flour	1½ cups
Buckwheat	⅞ cup
Soya flour	¼ cup

RECIPES

High Protein Wheat-Free Loaf

6 eggs, separated
1 tbsp sesame or caraway seeds
½ tsp salt
8 oz (200g) soya flour, sifted

1 Preheat oven to 180°C/350°F (Gas Mark 4).
2 Beat the egg yolks until very thick and pale. Add the seeds and salt.
3 Beat the egg whites until very stiff, then fold in the yolks. Add the flour to the mixture, carefully folding it all in.
4 Pour the mixture into a buttered 2.2 lb (1kg) loaf tin.
5 Bake for 25 minutes, then reduce the heat to 130°C/250°F (Gas Mark ½) and bake for a further 15 minutes.
6 Remove from the tin and cool on a wire rack.

Note: This bread is rather crumbly, with a fine sponge-like texture, but it is delicious toasted.

Egg, Wheat and Milk-Free Loaf

4 oz (100g) potato flour
4 oz (100g) buckwheat or soya flour
2 level tsps wheat-free baking powder
4 fl oz (125ml) water
1 tbsp oil
pinch of salt

1 Preheat oven to 200°C/400°F (Gas Mark 6).
2 Sieve together all dry ingredients.
3 Add water and oil.
4 Place mixture into a greased 1 lb (450g) bread tin and
  bake for 30–35 minutes.

Recommended Reading

Brostoff and Gamlin, *Food Allergy and Intolerance*, Bloomsbury, 1989

Randolf and Moss, *Allergies*, Turnstone Press, 1981

Rita Greer, *Wheat, Milk and Egg-Free Cooking*, Thorsons, 1995

C. Norman, *Recipes for Health: Migraine*, Thorsons, 1990

Maggie and Martin Budd, *Recipes for Health: Low Blood Sugar*, Thorsons, 1995

Martin L. Budd, *Low Blood Sugar*, Thorsons, 1995

Shirley Trickett, *Recipes for Health: Candida Albicans*, Thorsons, 1995

Rose and Gawell, *Migraine: The Facts*, Oxford University Press, 1981

T. N. Blau, *Migraine*, Chapman and Hall Medical, 1987

Turner and Simonsen, *Candida Albicans (Special Diet Cookbook)*, Thorsons, 1987

Leon Chaitow, *Candida Albicans*, Thorsons, 1985

Paavo Airola, *Hypoglycaemia – a Better Approach*, Health Plus Arizona, 1977

Hilda Cherry Hills, *Good Food To Fight Migraine*, Roberts Publications, 1979

Dr Mike Smith, *Migraine*, Kyle Cathie Ltd., 1994

Michelle Berriedale-Johnson, *Sainsbury's Special Diets Cookbook: Wheat-free, dairy-free, gluten-free, egg-free*, HarperCollins/Sainsbury's, 1995

Book Suppliers and Publishers

These specialists supply diet and health books:

- Merton Books, 24–26 High Street, Hampton Hill, Middlesex TW12 1PD. Tel: 0181 943 4244
- Books for Cooks, 4 Blenheim Crescent, London W11 1NN. Tel: 0171 221 1992
- Thorsons, HarperCollinsPublishers, 77–85 Fulham Palace Road, London W6 8JB. Tel: 0181 741 7070
- Berrydales' Special Diet Booklist, 5 Lawn Road, London NW3 2XS. Send an A5 stamped, self-addressed envelope plus £1.
- York Nutritional Laboratory, Tudor House, Lysander Close, Clifton Moor, York YO3 4XB. Tel: 01904 690640

Index